# Adventures with Jayce:

## Jayce's Big Surgery

Author: Jennifer Gaillard

Illustrator: Ebenezer Ogunbodede

## Dedications

This book is dedicated to everyone dear to me. My three lovely children, that inspire me every day. I do everything, because of you. My King, My husband, I love you very much. My nieces, my nephews, sisters, brothers, my mother Mary, my father Willie, my Aunt Betty Lou, and everyone close to me.

A special thank you to my best friend Kimberly. I don't know what I would do without you. My best cousins, Rosa, Whitney, and Sharlenna. Thank you to my friends LaSheena, Adria, and Miranda. Thank you, to my sister Willlette, for encouraging me to write. A very special Thank You to my Late Grandfather Tommy Burgess, for showing me how always encouraging me to be respectful and to do my best. I love you all.

ADVENTURES WITH JAYCE

My name is Jayce. I am six years old, and I am in the Kindergarten. I am the youngest of three children. My older sister's names are Mary and Terri. I love to ride my bicycle outside and I enjoy beating my drums.

A few weeks ago, my teacher gave me a note to give to my Mom. I am a pretty good reader but this note was in cursive writing, and I didn't understand how to read it. She gave me the note and said, "Here Jayce. This note is very important. Be sure to give it to your Mom." I said, "Yes ma'am. I sure will." When I got home, and I ran inside, threw my book bag down and went to my Mom's office. She's always there. She works from home, and told me to always be very quiet when I come in her office so I don't disturb her while she is working. I tiptoed in her office, I left the note on her desk. She gave me a thumbs up and then I walked out.

I made me a Peanut Butter and Jelly sandwich and poured a cold glass of milk. It was so good! After I finished my snack, I started on my homework.

A few minutes later, Mom got off of work, and sat on the chair beside me. The kitchen is where I enjoy working. That's what I do every day. I eat, and then I start working on my homework every day. I call that, my office.  She said, "Hey my favorite son!" "How was school today?" I laughed and answered "It was fine Mommy. I'm getting tired though and I want to take a nap." She said, "Ok, but be sure to finish up your homework." I said, "Yes ma'am".  That's how we talk in South Carolina. My Mom says, I'm supposed to answer all adults, "Sir or Ma'am" because that shows respect.

Mom had the note in her hand and opened it. She read it out loud and it said:

Hello,

I think Jayce has a bladder problem.

She said, "Hmm. Let me do some quick research and I'll be right back!"

I asked her, "Mommy, Mommy, What is a bladder problem". She said, "Remember how you said you have to keep going to the restroom all the time at school?" I said, "Yes". She said, "Well son, that's a bladder problem".

She went into her office and came out a few minutes later, and said, "Well Jayce, I made you a doctor's appointment" "The doctor is a specialist and she wants to make sure that everything is okay with you. I said, "Well Mommy, I don't think I need to go to a doctor's appointment for a bladder problem. Grandpa says he drinks Cranberry Juice, for his bladder problem." Mommy laughed and said, "Honey, this is a little different that Grandpas bladder. You know how he is, he likes to joke around. By the way, the doctor is going to just check out the situation, to see what we can do to get this all worked out". I told her "Well, I'm afraid to go". She grabbed my hand, and smiled, and said, "Don't be. The doctor will not hurt you, they want to make you feel better". I was still worried.  My sister Terri was in the Living Room, finishing up her homework. She likes to do her homework as soon as she gets home, so she can relax, for the rest of the day. She is two years older than me. She said, "Don't worry. You will be ok." I was sad and now getting mad because everyone is just saying "Don't worry". How could I not worry? I didn't want anything to be wrong with me. Why did my bladder have to have a problem?

I went in my room, and finished my homework. I laid down, but I was not sleepy anymore. I kept thinking and thinking and all of a sudden, I started to cry. I heard the house alarm go off, it said, "Front Door Open". Followed by a loud voice, "Hey Sweetheart" It was my Dad. He always calls mom Sweet Heart. I heard them talking and then right after that, he peeked in my door. "Hey Jay" "How's it going man?" my dad is the only person that calls me Jay. I said, "Not good. My bladder is broken and now I have to miss school to go to the doctor, for them to fix it. Grandpa said, the doctors only want to take your money and cause more problems" He started laughing and said, "No son, that's not true, Grandpa was only teasing. You don't have to be sad. You're a big boy and you've been to the doctor before. They've never hurt you before right?" "Right." I said. "Okay then, you should know, that this is only for the best. I know it seems scary and confusing, but you're not alone. We love you and you don't have to worry about going through this by yourself." He made me feel much better. He always know what to say to put a smile on my face. My Daddy is really tall, like a giant. He's not afraid of anything. So, if he's not afraid of a bladder problem, I'm not afraid of a bladder problem. I wiped my eyes and I gave him a big smile.

The next day, we were on our way to my doctor's appointment. Mom and I, got into her car, I buckled my seatbelt and I yelled to her, "Mommy, I'm all buckled!" "Good!" she said. Mommy always tell me, "Fasten your seat belt Jayce. An accident can happen at any time and I don't want to get cited for a ticket for breaking the law!" My mom stopped by a restaurant, she bought me my favorite breakfast, biscuit and gravy with and orange juice. It was delicious! After our breakfast we jumped back in the car, and were on our way again. I looked out the back window, at the buildings, wondering how long it was it was going to take us to get there. I thought about my friends at school, and wondered what they were learning. I loved to learn and I didn't want to miss out daily math review! That's my other favorite. Yes, math!

Mom stopped driving and I looked up, we were at a huge

building! Mom announced, "We're here!" She was excited but I wasn't. I said, "Mom, do I have to see the doctor?" She said, "Yes you do sweetie, you have to get checked out so that problem does escalates in to a bigger problem." I said, "Mom, what does escalates mean?" She said, "That's a big word for, out of control". She looked in her mirror and said "Cheer up! This is one of the best doctors ever! I did lots of research and she is excellent with children! She will take good care of you!" That made me feel better. Then I gave her a big smile. Then Mom said, "Now let's get inside before we are late for your appointment. Don't forget, be on your best behavior! No running around, no talking loud or playing in the doctor's office." "There may be little babies inside there asleep, and we don't want to disturb them!" I said, "OK Mommy. Yes, I don't want the little babies to start crying, so I'll be on my best behavior!"

We got out of the car and the wind was blowing very hard, it was very cold to. Luckily, I had on my new black jacket or I would have frozen. I put my hoody on my head and got a better sight of the building. WOW it was amazing! I was big, with bright colors. There was a gigantic train painted on the building, pictures of people, trees and lots of beautiful colors that I saw. (Purple, orange, green, yellow and my favorite color, blue!) It was so fun, that I started running inside! Mom yelled behind me, "Jayce! Wait on Mommy!" Then I stopped and waited on her.

I walked inside, and I saw lots of toys that I could play with! Blocks, choo choo trains, and books too! "Yes!" I whispered to myself. I asked, "Mommy, can I go play with the toys?" She said, "Yes, but use this hand sanitizer, afterwards because you don't

20

want to pick up any germs." She reached into her purse and got the hand sanitizer and handed it to me. I was used to that... Mommy is always talking about hand sanitizer and germs. She so scared of germs.

I sat down and had lots of fun, while Mommy signed my name at the front desk. My trip to the doctor was more fun than I thought it would be. There were other kids playing, pretty pictures and paintings on the wall, and everyone seemed so happy! Mommy sat down and chatted with another Mommy. She was holding a little baby. The baby, was wrapped in a yellow blanket. I remembered what Mommy told me.  I was sure to be quiet, and not to wake the sleeping babies. All of a sudden, I heard a ladies voice yell, "Jayce!" Suddenly, I stopped. All of the feelings of fear, rushed back to me at once! Mommy stood up and grabbed my hands. "Ok partner, that's us" The nurse was smiling with a blue jacket on, with lots of pictures on it to. She weighed me, checked my height and checked my temperature. Then she told us to follow her and we went in to a room.

The room was colorful too, with pictures of animals on the wall. The nurse said, "The Doctor with be with you shortly" then she closed the door.

The doctor came in the room. She smiled and shook my hand and said, "Hello, Jayce. My name is Dr. Jennifer. I'm your doctor,

and I will take care of you. I will
not hurt you and if I make you
feel uncomfortable, just let me
know". I giggled because she
was very nice and she had the
same name as my Mommy,
Jennifer. She pulled out some
pretty cool tools that she used
to check my health. Nothing
hurt and it was very fast.

The doctor told mommy that I
needed surgery. The doctor said,
"Jayce, the night before your
surgery, you cannot have any

24

food or drink after six pm. This is very important, ok?" I said, "Ok".

When I got to school, I told my teacher Ms. Johnson and my classmates, that I was having surgery. I let them know that I may miss school for a few days. They told me they would miss me to and my best friend Tyler even cried. I said to Tyler, "Don't cry, everything will be ok. I have to get surgery so that the problem doesn't escalate." I learned that word from Mommy.

My surgery was scheduled two days later, on Friday. When I got home from school, Thursday afternoon, the house smelled good. I could smell the food out of the door. Daddy, was in the kitchen cooking a big meal. I call my daddy, Bubba. I asked, "Bubba, umm. Something smells GOOD! What are you cooking?" He said, "Son, I'm cooking you favorite meal. Rice, cabbage, bar b que ribs and baked macaroni and cheese!" I opened my mouth wide. I was surprised! "Why are you cooking all that food?" He said "I wanted to make sure you eat a really good meal, before your surgery. I don't want my son to be hungry all night. "I ran up to him and gave him a big hug! I felt so special.

The food was so delicious. I even had seconds. I love to eat good food and my Daddy is the best cook I know. He loves to cook and cooks most of the food at home. Mommy, said, that is his job! When I get married, I want to be a great cook, just as him.

We had fun that night, we watched a movie and then I got ready for bed. I was not scared anymore. I said my prayers, and went to sleep.

Mom woke me up the next morning, I was still very sleepy. We walked outside, it was dark.

Mommy, Daddy, and my big sisters, all came with me to the hospital.

The hospital looked different than the doctor's office. There were no bright colors and pretty decorations there. Just plain white walls and pictures of trees, people in white coats and lots of other things. We got to our destination and waited. They called this area, the waiting room. We waited for a very long time and then finally, a nurse called my name. We all got up and followed her.

We walked down a long hallway, until we reached a room in the back of the building. I sat on the bed and put on a white and blue gown. I looked funny! The nurse gave me a yellow cap to go on my head and gave me some yellow matching socks, to go with it. A lot of doctors and nurses came, and told me who they were. I don't remember any of their names but they told me that they would take care of me.

Mommy and Daddy held my hand and they prayed with me and told me they would be waiting for me after my surgery.

The nurse gave me and I-Pad to play with. It was fun to! The doctor, came in and gave me some medicine, through a mask, and he called it gas.  I played with my I Pad and that's all.

The next thing I remember, was that I was at home! When I woke up, Mommy said, "Hello, Jayce. You did a great job, with your big surgery!"

She said, the medicine had me really sleepy and that's why I did not remember the ride home, from the hospital.

I stayed home for one week and I was sad because Mommy said, "Jayce, you cannot go outside and play, you have to wait until you feel better from your surgery". So I spent the entire week, watching television and reading fun books at home.

Over the weekend, my cousins Kaitlyn and Langston came to visit. Langston had a big brown Teddy Bear in his arm with a card in his hands. I was so happy when he gave it to me! He said, "This is for you Jayce. Mommy said you had surgery and we should buy you something special." Kaitlyn said, "What's up Jayce! How are you feeling?" I said, "I'm doing fine, just watching some TV." She said,

"That's good, I'm glad to hear that. Where's Mary?" She asked looking around the living room. I pointed to the room and said, "She's in her room, working on her cheer leading routine or something." She smiled and said, "Cool, I'm going to surprise her really quickly then. See ya later"". Then she walked away and went into Marys' room.

Mary is fourteen and Kaitlyns thirteen. They always hang out together. Kaitlyn comes over and they watch music videos and browse the internet on their I-Pads all day!

Langston said, "He Jayce, Lets go in your room, I want to play on your drums." "Sure" I said. He plays the drums at church so whenever he comes to visit, he always want to play my drum. He said he wants to be a famous drummer one day, and travel all over the world. I want to be famous to! I want to have my own television show and travel all over the world and cook like my Daddy. They will call me,

Chef Jayce! Chef Jayce the cooking man! Langston and I, went into my room. He didn't waste anytime getting on the drums. He beat those drums really loud! BOOM BOOM SNAP, BOOM BOOM SNAP! It sounded really well. I can't wait until I learn how to beat the drums like that! I was so happy to finally have a boy to play with! We played with my toy trucks, my Ninja Turtles and we even put together a puzzle. . We had lots of fun, and I forgot all about the surgery. Langston is so cool! We always have fun when we get together. He's in the 2$^{nd}$ grade and he teaches me all a lot about school. Plus, its good be around boys when you're around sisters all day! KNOCK KNOCK KNOCK. Langston got up and opened the door. I looked up and it was my Aunt Annette. I put on my sad face, hoping she would let my cousin's visit for a little longer. She said, "It's time to go Lang." (That's what she calls him for short) I said, please Aunt

Annette, I don't want Langston to leave yet. We just started playing." Annette said, "I know Jay, but we have to go because it's getting dark and we need to get on the road. I stood up and said, "OK Auntie Annette. Thank you for my gifts. I really appreciate it". She took her knuckles and gave me a little nudge on the head, and said, "you're welcome my little knuckle head." I gigged because she always call me that. That's why she is my favorite Auntie.

Then she asked, "Did you get a chance read the card that I gave you?" I said "No". She said, "Well read it then!" with a smile. I opened the card and $5 bill fell out. My eyes got wide! She surprised me. I said, "What? Money!" She laughed and said, "Put it in your piggy bank". I said, "Yes Ma'am!" I don't have a Piggy Bank but I hid it under my bed, in my old shoe box, where I have the rest of my money, until I get a new piggy bank. The old one broke last year when my friend Charlie came over. We were bouncing my basketball in my room and it hit my Piggy Bank. My sister Mary cleaned it up and my mom was upset because she told me before, "Do not play with the ball, in the house". So I guess, I learned my lesson.

I opened the card, and it read:

Dear Jayce

We love you and we hope you have a speedy recovery.

Love Langston and Family

We all hugged and then they left.

I placed my card on my dresser.

When Monday came, it was time to go to school again. I was so excited! When I back to school, everyone yelled, "JAYCE!" I tried not to smile that hard but I couldn't help it. I was so happy! Ms. Johnson and my classmates all ran up to me. The wanted to hug me but my teacher told them not to hug me to hard, because I just has surgery. I missed them too. All of the kids gathered around me and asked me questions about my surgery. I told them my experience. It was scary at first, but when you have people that show you love, it makes it easy to go through.

One month after my big surgery, I feel much better. It was a journey but hey, it wasn't that bad.  I feel great,   and I can go outside a play again

A Message from the Author

Thank you for reading this book. This is my first published book and I look for to bringing you great adventures and stories about my son Jayce.

# Contact Information

You may Email me at
Jennifer.Gaillard@yahoo.com

For Illustrations, or graphic designs, contact the illustrator at ebenezer4real01@yahoo.com

ADVENTURES WITH JAYCE

# Adventures with Jayce

# Jayce's Big Surgery